HOW TO CREATE A FLOURISHING FOOD FOREST

GROWING GREEN WITH SUSTAINABLE AND ECO-FRIENDLY FARMING TECHNIQUES

AVENTURAS DE VIAJE

Copyright SF Nonfiction Books © 2023

www.SFNonfictionBooks.com

All Rights Reserved

No part of this document may be reproduced without written consent from the author.

WARNINGS AND DISCLAIMERS

The information in this publication is made public for reference only.

Neither the author, publisher, nor anyone else involved in the production of this publication is responsible for how the reader uses the information or the result of his/her actions.

CONTENTS

Introduction   ix

Understanding Food Forest Principles   1
Assess and Analyze the Site   5
Set Your Goals   9
Design Your Food Forest   13
Develop a Planting Plan   18
Prepare the Soil   20
Start Planting   24
Observe and Adapt   26
Harvesting   29
Conclusion   32

Author Recommendations   35

THANKS FOR YOUR PURCHASE

Get Your Next SF Nonfiction Book FREE!

Claim the book of your choice at:

www.SFNonfictionBooks.com/Free-Book

You will also be among the first to know of all the latest releases, discount offers, bonus content, and more.

Go to:

www.SFNonfictionBooks.com/Free-Book

Thanks again for your support.

Get Your Next SF Nonfiction Book FREE!

Claim the book of your choice at:

www.SFNonfictionBooks.com

You will also be among the first to know of all the latest releases, discount offers, bonus content, and more.

Go to:

www.SFNonfictionBooks.com

Thanks again for your support.

INTRODUCTION

As environmental awareness and sustainability become a top priority in society, cultivating food that not only benefits us physically but also supports Earth health has become ever more essential.

Food forests offer an innovative and increasingly popular solution, which combines sustainable agricultural principles with nature's inherent wisdom to produce an abundant, diverse and self-sustenance source of nourishment. This book will lead you through every step of designing, planting and maintaining an edible forest.

It covers various aspects of food forest creation and management. Here is a snapshot of each chapter:

Understanding Food Forest Principles

In this chapter, we'll take an in-depth look at the fundamental principles that comprise food forests, including permaculture, agroforestry and the seven layers of a food forest. We will explore how these principles form the basis of a thriving and self-sustaining ecosystem.

Plan and Design Your Food Forest

You'll be guided through the process of selecting an ideal site, assessing climate/microclimate factors, managing water resources effectively and choosing appropriate plant species for your food forest.

Establishing Your Food Forest

We'll look at a range of planting techniques such as companion planting and polycultures as well as ways to create wildlife habitats which support natural pest control measures.

Maintaining a Thriving Food Forest

You'll gain practical tips for organic pest management, pruning and mulching procedures as well as water conservation to keep your food forest productive and thriving.

Harvest and Use Your Food Forest Bounty

Explore the proper timing, techniques, and methods of harvesting, preserving, storing, as well as exploring edible, medicinal and utilitarian uses for various plants in your Food Forest bounty.

Expanding Your Food Forest and Building Community

Discover ways to scale up your food forest by working with local organizations, teaching others about them and connecting multiple sites into an interlocking network of food forests for greater resilience within communities.

Case Studies and Success Stories

Gain inspiration from real-life food forest projects around the globe, learning from their best practices and lessons learned.

Conclusion

Explore how food forests could play an integral part in building a more eco-friendly world and your role as part of creating it.

Appendices

Gain valuable resources for further study with plant species lists and their applications; terminology glossaries; regional/climate specific recommendations and more!

Through this book, you will gain valuable insight into food forests and learn how to establish one that not only provides nourishment for both you and your community but also contributes to creating an eco-friendly future.

Whether an experienced gardener or a complete beginner, this comprehensive guide will equip you with all the knowledge you need to creating a flourishing food forest.

UNDERSTANDING FOOD FOREST PRINCIPLES

Before embarking on creating a flourishing food forest, it is necessary to understand its fundamental principles.

In this chapter we'll look at permaculture and agroforestry concepts as well as mimicking natural ecosystems for increased diversity and resilience benefits.

We will also take a peek are the seven layers that comprise food forests.

Permaculture and Agroforestry

Permaculture is a holistic design system that seeks to develop sustainable landscapes by merging human activities with nature in harmony. The system's three guiding ethics include Earth Care, People Care and Fair Share which emphasize the responsible use of resources by communities as well as equitable distribution of surplus resources.

Agroforestry is an ecological land management approach which integrates trees, shrubs and perennial plants with agricultural crops or livestock for optimal land usage, biodiversity enhancement and multiple benefits such as improved soil health, carbon sequestration and reduced erosion.

Food forests combine principles from both permaculture and agroforestry into one dynamic ecosystem that replicates its structure and function like any natural forest would do.

Mimicking Natural Ecosystems for Profit

Food forests seek to mimic the complex relationships and processes found within natural forest ecosystems by replicating them on an industrial scale. By doing this, their aim is largely self-sufficient;

needing minimal inputs for maintenance while producing multiple outputs from it.

An ecosystem in nature combines plants, animals, fungi and microorganisms in ways that create an interdependent balance and resilience that promotes its overall wellbeing. Such interactions include cycling nutrients through an ecosystem's food cycle; controlling pest populations with predatory insects and pollination of pollen-bearing flowers. By selecting and arranging plants in ways similar to nature's wisdom for food forest design, food forest designers can harness its inherent wisdom for more effective, productive, sustainable systems.

Biodiversity and Resilience in Sustainable Management Systems

Biodiversity is essential to creating a vibrant food forest, providing it with resilience and adaptability in response to pests, diseases, or changing climatic conditions. By including diverse plant species as well as wildlife populations within its borders, food forests can better withstand challenges caused by pests, diseases or weather shifts.

Resilience refers to a system's capacity to absorb disturbances while still functioning effectively, maintaining its basic structure and functions. Food forests increase resilience through using diverse plant species, encouraging healthy soil management practices, and creating supportive communities composed of plants, animals and microorganisms.

Food Forest Layers of Composition

Food forests should be designed to make efficient use of vertical space, much like natural forests do.

This typically happens by including seven distinct layers that contribute to overall productivity and diversity within their system:

Canopy Layer: Comprised of the tallest trees, this layer provides shade, habitat for wildlife and larger fruits and nuts for human consumption.

Sub-Canopy Layer: Comprising of smaller trees and large shrubs, this layer includes fruit- and nut-bearing species as well as nitrogen fixing species that help improve soil fertility.

Shrub Layer: This layer consists of smaller fruiting bushes, berry-producing plants and other shrubs which provide additional food and habitat for humans and wildlife alike.

Herbaceous Layer: This area comprises of culinary and medicinal herbs as well as plants which attract beneficial insects while discouraging pests from coming near it.

Groundcover Layer: Low-lying plants that spread horizontally make up this groundcover layer, helping to suppress weeds while conserving soil moisture levels and avoiding erosion.

Root Layer: The Root Layer includes edible roots, tubers and bulbs that grow beneath the soil's surface and contribute significantly towards breaking up compacted soil and improving overall structure of the environment. They play an essential part in breaking up compacted areas for improved soil structure.

Vertical Layer: Vines and other climbing plants form the vertical layer, taking advantage of vertical space while adding another dimension of productivity to food forests.

Through carefully selection of plants from each layer, a food forest can maximize its harvest, create an ecosystem rich in biodiversity and more efficiently utilize available space.

Understanding the principles that underlie the creation and management of a food forest is paramount for its success. By adopting concepts like permaculture and agroforestry, mimicking natural ecosystems, increasing biodiversity, resilience, and including all seven layers, you can build an agricultural system which will support itself while remaining eco-friendly - giving rise to self-sustenance, productivity, resilience and eco-friendliness all at the same time!

Keeping these guidelines in mind as you design and plan your very own food forest will yield you the best results.

ASSESS AND ANALYZE THE SITE

In this chapter, we will introduce site evaluation and analysis as an integral step toward creating a food forest. This step provides essential data necessary for informed plant selection decisions, design choices and management decisions.

In particular, climate, topography, soil composition and moisture availability along with any existing vegetation on-site.

Climate

Understanding your site's climate is paramount when creating a food forest; this determines which plants will flourish there and should be carefully considered during the selection phase.

Hardiness Zones

Determine your hardiness zone by taking note of the average annual minimum temperature in your region and measuring it on an hour-by-hour basis. Having this information handy can assist when selecting plants suitable for cold tolerance in your locale.

Precipitation

Analyzing average annual precipitation and rainfall distribution throughout the year in your area will allow you to select plants which thrive with available water sources while devising appropriate water management strategies.

Temperature and Seasonal Variations

To select plants suited to the temperature range in your region and harvest at optimal times, keep track of average high and low temperatures as well as any drastic shifts. This information can help you choose those with adaptable roots while making decisions regarding when planting and harvesting should occur.

Topography

Assess your site to understand how its topographical elements might impede water, air and sunlight flow.

Slope

Consider how the slope and aspect of your site affect water runoff, erosion and solar exposure. South-facing slopes tend to see more sunshine while north-facing ones remain cooler and shaded by surrounding structures.

Elevation

Make note of any elevation differences within your food forest that might create microclimates to support plant diversity. Take note of any elevation shifts which might offer opportunities for microclimate manipulation when cultivating plants within this environment.

Landforms

Landforms such as hills, valleys or depressions could influence water flow patterns or offer unique growing conditions. It is crucial to pay close attention to these things.

Soil

Achieving food forest success starts with healthy soil. Assess the suitability of your soil for plant growth and make any needed amendments.

Soil Texture

Examining your soil texture will enable an accurate evaluation of drainage, water-holding capacity and nutrient availability.

Soil Structure

The arrangement of soil particles has an effect on aeration, drainage and root penetration. Investigate this.

pH Level

By conducting a soil pH test you can determine both nutrient availability and plant growth. Most plants prefer an acidic to neutral pH (6.0-7.0).

Soil Nutrients

Analyzing soil nutrients such as nitrogen, phosphorus and potassium will allow you to make informed choices when selecting suitable plant species and managing fertility issues in the soil.

Informed decisions will assist you with planting purposes as well as increasing overall plant productivity.

Water

Food forests rely heavily on their water sources for survival, and you should assess both availability and quality to create an effective management plan.

Water Sources

Locate natural water sources such as streams, ponds or springs, and evaluate their quality and reliability.

Rainwater Harvesting

Evaluate your potential rainwater harvesting capabilities according to the size and composition of your catchment area (i.e. roofs or pavement) as well as average annual precipitation amounts.

Irrigation

Assess whether irrigation is needed and take steps to learn about and decide what is best for your needs. Consider drip systems, sprinklers and flood systems.

Existing Vegetation

Inspection of existing vegetation on your site can provide invaluable insights into its history, soil health and potential plant growth potential. Incorporation of existing plants can even be part of your food forest design plan.

Plant Inventory

Take inventory of existing species found within your food forest such as trees, shrubs and herbaceous. Make note of any species which could become invasive, diseased or detrimental in future years.

Plant Health

Evaluate the overall health of existing vegetation to assess soil fertility, water availability, and any pest/disease concerns.

Succession

Pay close attention to the stages of plant succession on your site as this can provide valuable insight into natural processes at work, which in turn will inform your food forest design.

Wildlife

Be wary of any wildlife present that might impede your food forest's success as an edible landscape, including beneficial species like pollinators and natural predators as well as herbivores or pests that might threaten its viability.

Conclusion

Proper assessment and analysis are vital elements in creating an eco-friendly food forest that will thrive. By understanding each site individually, you can make more informed decisions regarding plant selection, design, management practices and maintenance that ensure its survival.

SET YOUR GOALS

Before undertaking the design and implementation of your food forest, it's crucial to set specific, well-defined goals. These goals will act as the cornerstone for the project as you make informed decisions along the way.

In this chapter we will cover the significance of goal setting as well as factors to keep in mind when setting those goals, along with advice for developing specific, achievable, measurable objectives for your food forest project.

Why Establish Goals for Your Food Forest?

Setting goals for your food forest is integral for numerous reasons.

Clear Direction

Setting specific goals helps keep you focused on what it is you wish to accomplish, making sure all efforts are directed toward meeting desired outcomes.

Decision-Making

Goals provide a roadmap for making sound decisions when planning, designing and overseeing your food forest project.

Motivation

Knowing your objectives helps you to move towards accomplishing them even when challenges present themselves.

Evaluation

By setting measurable goals, it will allow you to track the progression and assess the success of your food forest over time.

Factors to Keep In Mind When Setting Goals

Setting goals for your food forest involves considering several essential aspects.

Personal Needs and Values

Before creating a food forest, evaluate why it's important for you to do so - are your intentions focused on feeding yourself or others, creating space for relaxation or increasing biodiversity?

Your personal needs and values are the keystones of your goals.

Site Characteristics

Carefully evaluate the characteristics of your site, such as size, topography, climate and existing vegetation - they all affect what types of plants can be grown as part of a food forest and how best it should be designed.

Time and Resources

Set realistic expectations regarding how much time, effort, and resources can be dedicated to your project. Your goals should remain achievable while considering all available resources.

Community and Ecosystem Benefits

Assess how this food forest project might have wider ramifications on both local ecosystems as well as the community itself, such as improved water quality, habitat creation or social engagement initiatives.

Establishing Goals That Can Be Met and Measured

Once you have taken into account all the above considerations, the next step should be setting specific, achievable and measurable goals for your food forest.

Be Specific

Be clear in what your goals for your food forest are. Rather than setting broad-brush goals like "grow food," strive towards something specific such as "growing enough fruits and vegetables to provide my family of four with enough nourishment throughout the year".

Break It Down

Break down your goals into more manageable targets and objectives, for example "attract pollinators and create habitat for native birds".

Be Realistic

Establish goals that are realistic given your site characteristics, time commitment and resources available. Starting small can often prove more successful than setting overly ambitious goals that lead to disappointment later.

Establish Measurable Criteria

Develop criteria to measure the success of your goals in a way that allows you to track their progression and adjust as necessary. For example, if your aim is to enhance soil fertility you might measure soil organic matter levels before and after creating your food forest.

Set Timeframes

Create deadlines to stay on course and maintain momentum towards reaching your goals and objectives. Doing this can keep you accountable and moving in the right direction.

Example Goals for a Food Forest

Here are a few examples to consider when creating your own food forest goals.

- Produce 70% of our family's annual fruit and vegetable needs within three years, by creating a multi-layered food forest of at least 50 edible plant species.

- Attract and support pollinators by planting at least 10 species of flowering plants that provide nesting sites, while decreasing water consumption by 50% within three years through water-saving techniques and drought-tolerant planting options.
- Provide habitat for native birds and wildlife by including native plant species into nesting and foraging sites. Set up a community education program within two years for sharing knowledge and skills associated with sustainable food production.

With your goals clearly laid out, you have taken an essential first step toward realizing your vision of an expansive food forest.

Remember, goal setting is an ongoing process and as your experience and knowledge increase, so may the need to alter or modify them.

DESIGN YOUR FOOD FOREST

A food forest is a self-sustaining, eco-friendly, and multi-layered ecosystem designed to mimic the natural structure and function of a forest. By implementing principles of permaculture and sustainable agriculture, a food forest provides a diverse array of edible plants, including fruits, nuts, herbs, and vegetables.

In this chapter, we'll guide you through the process of designing your own food forest, taking into account factors such as climate, soil, water availability, and plant selection.

Site Assessment and Climate Considerations

Step one in designing your food forest should involve an assessment of its site and understanding of local climate.

Sunlight

Determine the sunniest areas on your site as fruit and nut trees require full sun exposure for best growth.

Water Availability

Investigate natural water sources and drainage patterns as well as potential areas for rainwater harvesting.

Soil Quality

To accurately gauge soil quality, conduct soil tests to ascertain pH, nutrient levels and texture.

Wind Exposure

Plant windbreaks to shield your food forest from strong winds.

Climate

It is important to understand your region's climate in order to select plants appropriate for its hardiness zone.

Plant Selection and Placement

Choose a diverse range of plants that provide food, habitat, and other ecosystem services.

Climate Suitability

Check that plants are suitable for your hardiness zone and microclimate before planting.

Pollination

Plant both self-pollinating and cross-pollinating species to increase pollination efficiency for fruit set success.

Pest Control

Include plants that deter pests while simultaneously drawing in beneficial insects or birds that feed on them as part of your strategy for controlling them.

Nitrogen-fixing plants

Legumes such as beans and peas can help increase soil fertility.

When placing plants, consider growth habits, lighting needs and root patterns. Arrange them so that their features complement one another for maximum space utilization and mutually beneficial relationships - such as planting sun-loving species near the southern side of a food forest and shade-tolerant species in the understory.

Water and Irrigation

Design your food forest to efficiently capture and store water resources.

Swales

Contoured trenches that slow, spread and sink water into the landscape.

Rainwater harvesting

Collect and store rainwater from rooftops or other surfaces before using it later for reuse in other ways.

Mulching

Apply an organic layer around plants to help conserve soil moisture levels and help retain it for plant health.

Drip irrigation

Install a water-efficient irrigation system to minimize water waste.

Maintenance and Monitoring

Food forests are designed to require little care; however, regular tasks will still need to be performed.

Pruning

Prune trees and shrubs to maintain their health, increase yield, and ensure good airflow.

Mulching

Refresh mulch around plants as necessary to conserve soil moisture and suppress weeds.

Pest Management

Monitor for pests and diseases to apply organic controls when necessary.

Fertility Management

Apply compost or other organic amendments to maintain soil fertility.

Harvest

Harvest fruits, nuts, and other produce regularly in order to foster further production.

At each step of the food forest's development, it's essential to monitor and make necessary changes as needed. Keep an eye out on how plants interact and perform, then alter your design based on those observations. Over time, your food forest will become self-sustainable as plants mature and form beneficial relationships among each other.

Perennial Polycultures

The use of perennial polycultures, which are diverse plantings of long-lived species, is an integral component of food forest design. Perennial polycultures offer several advantages over their food forest counterparts.

Improved Productivity

Polycultures have proven more productive at producing food throughout the year, creating a consistent harvest.

Resilience

With less exposure to pests, diseases, and climate extremes than monocultures, resilience of polycultures increases substantially.

Soil Health

Planting an array of species with differing root depths and growth habits can significantly enhance soil structure, fertility, and water retention.

In order to design an effective perennial polyculture, take into account these guidelines:

Complementary Functions

Select plants that provide multiple benefits, such as food production, pest control or nitrogen fixation.

Spatial Arranging

Arrange plants to maximize space and sunlight availability so each one may thrive and flourish.

Succession

Plant species which mature at various times to ensure a continuous harvest cycle.

Planning and cultivating a food forest can be an exhilarating and creative journey. By selecting and placing plants strategically, you can foster beneficial relationships among them while optimizing their output. With proper care and maintenance, your food forest should produce abundant harvests while simultaneously supporting wildlife in its region.

DEVELOP A PLANTING PLAN

A planting plan serves as the blueprint for organizing and placing various plant species throughout your food forest. It is extremely important in order to give your forrest the best chance of success.

Create a Planting Map

Once you have chosen your plant species and organized them into guilds, create a planting map. The planting map outlines where each plant should go in your food forest.

- Space your plants appropriately to avoid overcrowding and competition for resources.
- Plant in layers for maximum space utilization and to form a multi-dimensional ecosystem.
- Optimize light exposure by placing taller plants to the north side while smaller ones to the south side.
- Consider ease of access and maintenance when placing plants

Implement and Maintain Your Planting Plan

Now that your planting plan is in place, it's time to implement and maintain it. Prepare the site, source healthy plants from local nurseries, and install them according to your map. After planting, monitor its progress and health closely so as to make adjustments as needed; regular maintenance tasks could include:

- Watering and irrigation
- Mulching and composting
- Pruning and thinning
- Pest and disease management

Establishing a planting plan is key to creating a flourishing food forest. By understanding your site, selecting appropriate plant species, organizing them into guilds, and creating a planting map you can maximize health, productivity, and sustainability.

Careful planning, ongoing monitoring and regular maintenance will allow your food forest to flourish as an interconnected ecosystem.

PREPARE THE SOIL

An effective food forest depends on rich, fertile soil that's full of life. Soil preparation is the cornerstone of creating a productive and sustainable ecosystem.

In this chapter we'll go through various techniques for prepping soil before planting your food forest.

Assess Your Soil Type

Step one is identifying your soil type. Soil types vary in terms of texture, drainage, and nutrient content - with three primary categories including sand, silt, and clay. An ideal food forest soil will be a loamy blend made up of all three.

You can perform a simple jar test or consult with local soil testing labs in order to ascertain your individual soil composition and levels of nutrition.

Amend the Soil

Based on the results of your soil test, you may need to amend it in order to create an ideal environment for your plants.

Compost

Organic matter is vital to soil fertility. By adding well-aged compost into your soil, you'll increase its nutrient content, aeration and water retention capabilities.

Sand

Sand can improve drainage and airflow if your soil contains heavy clay content; using it may increase drainage as well.

Clay

By adding clay to sandy soils, you can increase water retention and nutrient-holding capacity.

Lime

If your soil has too much acidity, adding lime may help balance its pH level.

Remember to only add amendments in moderation as too much can cause imbalance and poor soil conditions.

Build Your Soil's Microbial Life

An active microbial community is essential for maintaining a sustainable food forest. Microorganisms play an essential role in breaking down organic matter, providing vital nutrients to support plant growth, and encouraging root development.

Mulch

Spreading an organic mulch such as wood chips or straw over your soil helps retain moisture, regulate temperatures and stimulate microbial activity in your garden.

No-Till

To preserve soil structure and the ecosystem, avoid tilling. Tilling your soil can destroy its structure and disrupt the microbial ecosystem. Instead, loosen it gently with a broadfork or other similar tool.

Plant Cover Crops

Clover, vetch or rye can all be grown as cover crops that will eventually be integrated back into the soil to add organic material and draw in beneficial microbes.

Create Soil Layers

Mimicking the natural layers found in forests is essential to creating an effective food forest. By creating distinct soil layers, you will maximize water and nutrient use.

Topsoil

Your soil's top layer should consist of nutrient-rich, well-draining soil that's filled with organic matter for proper drainage.

Subsoil

The layer beneath your topsoil should have looser structure to allow deeper root penetration and water infiltration.

Deep Soil

Your deepest layer of soil should be the densest and most compact, acting as an underground reservoir for water and nutrients.

Address Drainage Issues

Proper drainage is crucial to creating a successful food forest. Waterlogged soil can suffocate plant roots and encourage fungal diseases. If your soil drains poorly, consider one or more of the following solutions.

Swales

These trenches should be dug with shallow, gently sloping trenches that slope away from planting areas in order to redirect excess water away.

Raised Beds

Raising planting areas above grade is another effective way of improving drainage and aeration.

French Drains

Install perforated pipes surrounded by gravel to redirect excess water away.

Preparing the soil for your food forest requires careful and deliberate consideration. By assessing your soil type, amending as necessary, encouraging microbial life, creating layers, and addressing drainage issues, you can create the ideal foundation for a thriving eco-friendly food forest.

START PLANTING

Previous chapters explored the importance of planning, designing, and preparing your site for your food forest. Now that your foundation is firm, it is time to get planting!

Planting Techniques

Digging Holes

For trees and large shrubs, dig holes at least twice the width and depth of their root balls and root systems. Fill the hole partially with water before placing the plant to ensure proper root-to-soil contact.

Sheet Mulching

This technique can be utilized for growing ground cover plants, herbs, and other small plants in an easy and cost-effective manner.

Start by spreading out a layer of cardboard or newspaper over the area where you wish to plant in order to suppress weeds while maintaining moisture.

Cover this cardboard with compost then plant directly into it; as cardboard breaks down over time it provides additional nutrients into your soil.

Companion Planting

Companion planting is essential to creating a thriving ecosystem, as it involves planting various species together that have mutually beneficial relationships.

An example would be planting legumes near fruit trees to provide nitrogen or planting flowers with pollinators-attracting pollen or predatory insects to control pests.

Mulching and Watering

Once your plants are in the ground, it's crucial that they receive proper care and attention. Mulching with organic materials like wood chips, straw or leaves is an effective way to retain moisture, suppress weeds and regulate soil temperatures while providing sufficient hydration to develop strong root systems.

Ongoing Maintenance

To ensure the long-term success of your food forest, be prepared to devote both time and effort in its ongoing care. This includes pruning, watering, pest management and disease control.

You can also consider thinning out certain plants to reduce competition. This will help maintain a healthy, productive ecosystem.

OBSERVE AND ADAPT

As you embark on the path toward creating a flourishing food forest, it is crucial to develop an attitude of continuous learning and adaptation. Nature is dynamic; your food forest should mirror this change. In this chapter we will examine how observation and adaptation play an integral part in building sustainable, eco-friendly food forests.

Observe the Landscape

Before planning your food forest, take time to observe its natural patterns. Take note of aspects like sunlight exposure, water availability, soil quality and wildlife presence - this will allow you to design an edible landscape that works seamlessly within its surroundings.

Learn from Nature

Eco-friendly farming involves imitating natural ecosystems. You should research their patterns, relationships and functions before applying them to your food forest. Study how plants grow in nature - their interactions with other plants as well as adaption to their environment - in order to design an eco-friendly system which is both productive and resilient.

Monitor Your Progress

Regular observations of your food forest are crucial for making informed decisions. Take note of how plants respond to changes in their environment such as weather fluctuations, pest infestations or disease outbreaks. monitor the growth and health of your plants, and pay attention to any unexpected changes. This will allow you to spot potential issues early and address them before they deteriorate further.

Experiment and Adapt

As your food forest matures, don't be afraid to explore new techniques or combinations for plants. By testing different approaches and monitoring their success over time, you may gain invaluable insights that help enhance and develop it further.

Foster Diversity

Diverse food forests are more resilient to pest outbreaks or disease than monoculture systems. Encourage biodiversity by planting native and perennial crop species as well as those that are pollinator-friendly. Not only will this create an effective food forest system but it will also provide shelter for beneficial insects and wildlife that live there.

Embrace Change

As your food forest matures, its needs and conditions will change over time. Be ready to adjust your management practices accordingly - for instance, by thinning out some trees to allow more sunlight into the forest floor, or changing the watering schedule to meet changing plant demands. Being open and flexible with change will ensure a thriving and adaptable food forest.

Learn from Others

Take comfort knowing you are not alone on your quest to build a thriving food forest. Find fellow farmers, gardeners, and permaculture practitioners to share knowledge and experiences. Attend workshops, conferences, or local gatherings where successful and unsuccessful food forest initiatives are presented as examples. Also, be open to receiving feedback on your own efforts from peers.

At its core, creating a successful food forest lies in carefully monitoring and responding to its ever-evolving environment. By being open to experimentation and change in your food forest and closely overseeing it yourself, you will create a sustainable ecosystem that offers abundant food sources while supporting local wildlife populations and contributing to a healthier planet.

HARVESTING

In previous chapters, we explored how to establish and grow a vibrant food forest from scratch using eco-friendly farming techniques that emphasize sustainability and growth.

Now it's time to reap your labor's rewards by harvesting its bounty!

In this chapter we will cover essential techniques, tips and best practices for harvesting your food forest in order to guarantee a continuous supply of fresh produce while upholding its integrity and sustainability.

Harvesting Techniques and Timing

Timing is of utmost importance when harvesting produce. Collecting too early could result in underdeveloped or unripe fruits and vegetables, while waiting too long could result in spoilage or loss of vital nutrients. Here are some guidelines to follow:

- Examine Your Plants: Pay close attention to the color, texture and scent of your fruits and vegetables. Become acquainted with their ideal appearance when harvest time arrives.
- Taste Test: In order to properly evaluate fruits, it's vitally important to taste them at various stages of ripeness to determine when is the optimal time for harvesting.
- Track Ripening: Maintain a journal to record changes in appearance, flavor and overall quality over time. This will help determine the best time to harvest in future years.
- Staggered Harvesting: Staggering the harvesting of plants or species over time can extend their harvest period and ensure you always have access to fresh produce.

Selective Harvesting

Selective harvesting is an efficient technique used to harvest only the ripest or most mature fruits and vegetables from your plants while leaving other produce to continue maturing naturally. This practice maintains healthy plants, reduces waste, and ensures produce of superior quality.

- Harvest only what you need: Avoid over-harvesting so your food forest continues producing long into the future.
- Leave some fruits and vegetables behind: Allow some fruits and vegetables to remain on plants as habitat and food for wildlife while simultaneously increasing biodiversity.
- Rotate Your Harvests: Try harvesting different areas and plants each time, giving the others time to recover and produce even more food. This way, your forest won't become overgrown with harvest debris.

Proper Harvesting Tools

Selecting appropriate tools for harvesting is key to making the process more effective. It also protects plants from damage and prolongs productivity.

Hand pruners are ideal for harvesting fruits, vegetables and herbs attached by stems from their respective plants.

A harvesting knife is convenient when cutting through thick stems such as those found on squash or melons vines.

Fruit pickers are long-handled tools fitted with baskets or claws at their ends that make for easy fruit picking in high places.

Gardner gloves will protect your hands against cuts, thorns and dirt while handling plants and produce.

A harvesting basket is useful to store all those newly picked fruits and veggies.

Post-Harvest Handling and Storage

Post-harvest handling and storage practices are essential to the quality and freshness of produce.

Ensure everything is clean and dry. Gently rinse your produce in water to remove dirt or debris before leaving it to air dry naturally.

Arrange produce by type before storing accordingly - some fruits and vegetables produce ethylene gas which hastens ripening processes in other items in your storeroom.

Freeze, can, or dry any excess produce so that it may be enjoyed all year.

Disperse your bounty among friends and family or donate it to local food banks as a way to reduce waste while supporting community engagement.

Harvesting is the satisfying reward for all of your hard work in creating a flourishing food forest. By following the techniques and best practices outlined here, harvesting can provide a consistent source of fresh, nutritious, eco-friendly produce.

CONCLUSION

Together, we have explored the fascinating world of food forests. From their principles to site analysis, goal setting, design, planting and adaptation through to harvesting.

My aim has been to equip you with all of the knowledge, skills and strategies necessary for you to create your own food forest and contribute to global efforts of ecological restoration and sustainable living.

As we near the conclusion of this guide, it's essential that we remember the significance of what we're undertaking. Establishing a food forest is much more than an indulgent hobby or source of fresh produce; it represents resilience, commitment to harmonious co-existence with nature and an initiative for leaving a greener, healthier planet behind for future generations.

Food forests start with one seed: an infinitely small piece of potential. As it takes shape, however, a web of life emerges as various species, each playing their unique roles, collaborate and compete to form an intricate network. While it may require patience at times and additional weeding efforts may be necessary; once complete you will reap many rewards. An abundant source of nutritious food will become available as well as biodiversity enhancement, soil health improvement, and providing habitats for numerous forms of life.

As you embark on your food forest-building journey, keep this in mind: both its process and end product are equally significant. Each food forest is different due to the specifics of its site, the goals of its creator and the constant interaction between these factors. Expect surprises and be prepared to adapt. Some of the greatest lessons are learned through trial-and-error experiences; remain flexible and open-minded throughout your endeavor.

Food forests should not only produce, but also contribute positively to their surrounding ecosystem by supporting biodiversity and enriching the lives of those who interact with it. Successful food forests must not just be sustainable but regenerative - giving back more to the earth than they take from it.

Let this book serve as your starting point, guide and inspiration; however, your true masterclass lies within nature itself - in its soil beneath your feet, its plants around you and sky overhead - where profound teachings await. Take this chance to learn, grow and create something truly meaningful!

Remember, you aren't simply planting trees; you are planting the future! I wish you all the best on this exciting, enriching, and transformative journey as you make our Earth greener one food forest at a time.

Dear reader,

Thank you for reading *How to Create a Flourishing Food Forest*.

If you enjoyed this book, please leave a review where you bought it. It helps more than most people think.

Don't forget your FREE book!

You will also be among the first to know of FREE review copies, discount offers, bonus content, and more.

Go to:

www.SFNonfictionBooks.com

Thanks again for your support.

AUTHOR RECOMMENDATIONS

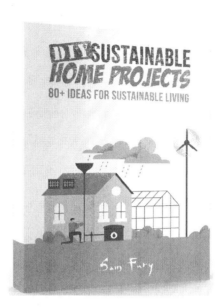

Discover 80+ Sustainable Living Projects

Start making your home more sustainable today, because this book has DIY projects for everyone.

Get it Free Today

www.SFNonfictionBooks.com/diy-sustainable-home-projects

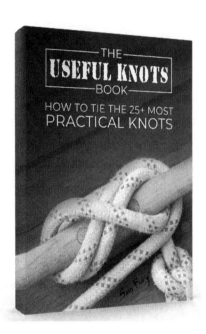

Discover the Only Knots You'll Ever Need!

Learn how to tie the only knots you'll ever need, because this book has the 25 most practical knots there are.

Get it Free Today

www.SFNonfictionBooks.com/the-useful-knots-book

Printed in Great Britain
by Amazon